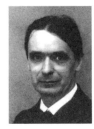 RUDOLF STEINER (1861–1925) called his spiritual philosophy 'anthroposophy', meaning 'wisdom of the human being'. As a highly developed seer, he based his work on direct knowledge and perception of spiritual dimensions. He initiated a modern and universal 'science of spirit', accessible to anyone willing to exercise clear and unprejudiced thinking.

From his spiritual investigations Steiner provided suggestions for the renewal of many activities, including education (both general and special), agriculture, medicine, economics, architecture, science, philosophy, religion and the arts. Today there are thousands of schools, clinics, farms and other organizations involved in practical work based on his principles. His many published works feature his research into the spiritual nature of the human being, the evolution of the world and humanity, and methods of personal development. Steiner wrote some 30 books and delivered over 6000 lectures across Europe. In 1924 he founded the General Anthroposophical Society, which today has branches throughout the world.

Rudolf Steiner was not concerned with systems. His aim was to suggest impulses towards finding and developing ways of living that would be worthy of humanity in the here and now. One aspect of this was his wish to intensify our awareness of existence as something that is not limited to our present life between birth and death. He never tired of reminding us that we are in reality spiritual entities. Through his written works and lectures Steiner urged us to take this hidden reality seriously, encouraging us in countless ways to develop an awareness of spirituality—a presence of mind that would enable us to recognize and do what is necessary in any given moment. Yet when faced with the voluminous dimensions of his work, it is easy to lose sight of this.

*The '**spiritual perspectives**' presented in this series assemble core ideas on specific subjects, as found in his complete works, with the aim of bringing mobility into thinking while also deepening the ability to understand and act. The brief extracts do not claim to provide exhaustive treatment of a subject. Their purpose is to open up approaches to the prodigious complex of Steiner's work, so as to assist readers as they endeavour to gain their own understanding of his extraordinary world of ideas.*

The source references are intended to serve as initial signposts. However, some will find the fragments sufficient in themselves—as valuable aids to making one's way in the complex world that surrounds us.

ON EPIDEMICS

spiritual perspectives

RUDOLF STEINER

compiled and edited by Taja Gut
translated by J. Collis

RUDOLF STEINER PRESS

Rudolf Steiner Press
Hillside House, The Square
Forest Row, RH18 5ES

www.rudolfsteinerpress.com

Published by Rudolf Steiner Press 2011

Originally published in German under the title *Stichwort Epidemien* by
Rudolf Steiner Verlag, Dornach, in 2010. This authorized translation is
published by permission of the Rudolf Steiner Nachlassverwaltung,
Dornach

A catalogue record for this book is available from the British Library

ISBN: 978 1 85584 262 5

Cover by Andrew Morgan Design
Typeset by DP Photosetting, Neath, West Glamorgan
Printed and bound by Gutenberg Press, Malta

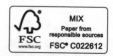

MIX
Paper from
responsible sources
FSC
www.fsc.org   FSC® C022612

CONTENTS

1. EPIDEMICS AND INFECTION

Every human being is an individual

The profoundest and most significant principle is that we must view the individuality of the human being as a unique reality which is utterly different from that of any other human being.[1]

Fear of bacteria

It is maintained—and perhaps not without a degree of justification, or with some degree of one-sided justification—that orthodox medicine has created a real fear of bacteria.[*] On the other hand, however, investigations have shown that the overall health of the population has improved in recent decades. Advocates of this view point proudly to the percentage reduction in mortality rates in one place or another over the decades. But then there are also those who maintain that it is not so much a matter of considering external circumstances with regard to ill health; for them the causes which lie within individual human beings are what matter, their proclivity for certain conditions or whether their lifestyle is sensible or foolish. These people are more likely to point out that while the mortality rate has undeniably declined in recent times there is nevertheless a shocking

---

[*] Viruses were not discovered until around 1890, and in Steiner's day there was as yet little talk of viruses among the wider population. In the texts quoted here the word 'bacterium' refers not only to bacteria but also to all micro-organisms that cause diseases, including viruses.

increase in the number of people who are ill. They emphasize the increase in certain specific forms of illness: heart diseases, cancers, illnesses that never used to be mentioned in medical literature, diseases of the digestive organs, and so on. Of course the reasons given by both the one side and the other must be taken seriously. From a superficial point of view it cannot be denied that bacteria are the most terrible causes of disease. But on the other hand there is also no denying that individuals are either resistant to the causes of disease or they are not. They are not resistant if they have destroyed their ability to resist through living an inappropriate lifestyle.[2]

In olden times people thought illnesses came from God; nowadays they are said to come from bacteria

How can we distinguish between an illness that can be accounted for by external circumstances and an illness for which the whole cause lies within the human organism in a way that makes us think that it has come of its own accord without any external cause? Well, things are not quite so simple. Nevertheless we are justified in saying that illnesses can occur for which a person may be particularly susceptible on account of his inner disposition. On the other hand, though, there are also many symptoms for which external causes can be discerned. For example if we break a leg we have to take external circumstances into account, although there may be other reasons as well. And the same goes for accidents caused by the weather. Conditions in city slums can also to some extent be regarded as external causes. The possibilities are manifold. It is easy to understand why the modern trend in medicine is to see illnesses as having been caused by external circumstances, especially bacteria. Indeed this has gone so far that one individual with a sense of humour has declared, not without justification: Nowadays illnesses come from bacteria just as in days gone by it was said that they came from God or the devil. In the thirteenth century people said that illnesses came from God, and in the fifteenth century they said they came from the devil. Later still they thought that the humours were the cause, and nowadays they are the result of bacteria. Thus have people's views supplanted one another over the ages.[3]

Fears conform to popular trends

The fear to which people succumb nowadays closely resembles the medieval fear of ghosts: this is our present fear of bacteria. These two states of fear are objectively the same. Ideas during the Middle Ages were in keeping with their time just as our ideas nowadays befit our time. People in medieval times had some belief in the spiritual world and so of course they had a fear of spiritual beings. In modern times we no longer believe in the spiritual world, so our fear is directed towards physical beings, be they ever so small.[4]

Dependence on authority, dread of ghosts and fear of bacteria

Whatever the age in which one lives, one must be especially sceptical in respect of the authority prevalent in that age. Without spiritual insight one can make serious mistakes in this regard.

This is especially the case in one particular field of human culture, namely in the field of materialistic medicine. Here we can see clearly how there is increasing dependence upon whatever those in authority consider to be the standard, so that far more dreadful things can result nowadays than were brought about by the much maligned authorities of the Middle Ages. We are in the midst of this already, and it will become ever more pronounced. When people mock the medieval belief in ghosts one can but ask: 'Are things any different today? Is there any less fear of ghosts nowadays? Are not people afraid of many more ghosts now than they were then?'

Things are far worse now than anyone can imagine. Think what must be going on in the human soul when we are told: 'There, in the palm of your hand, you have 60,000 bacteria!' Scientists in America have calculated the number of bacteria present in a single moustache. Surely such a thing ought to persuade us to say: Those medieval ghosts were at least respectable ghosts; but today's bacterial ghosts are altogether too diminutive, too unsuitable to be regarded with such fear, especially as this fear is now only in its early stages, for it will lead to a dependence on authority in the field of health which will be truly dire.[5]

Bacteria are most intensively nurtured by a materialistic mind set

Today we shall be dealing with the fact that bacteria can only become dangerous when they are nurtured and cherished . . . Bacteria are most intensively nurtured when human beings take nothing but materialistic thoughts with them upon entering into the state of sleep. The best way to nurture bacteria is to enter into sleep with nothing but materialistic ideas in mind. From out of the spiritual world the 'I' and the astral body then work down into the organs of the physical body which are neither the blood nor the nervous system. Going to sleep in a materialistic frame of mind is the very best way to nurture bacteria.[6]

Fear of epidemics provides the best habitat for bacteria
Actually there is at least one other means that is as effective: to live within a seat of epidemic or endemic diseases and to absorb only the case histories by which one is surrounded while being entirely filled with a sense of dread concerning these illnesses. This is just as effective. If we can bring nothing up out of ourselves except fear of the illnesses which surround us at the seat of an epidemic, and if we go to sleep at night filled with nothing but thoughts of this fear, then we create unconscious replicas, imaginations, which are drenched in fear. And this is an excellent method for nurturing bacteria. But if we can reduce this fear even by a small amount in our everyday work, if, for example, in caring for the patients, we can forget that there might be a danger of becoming infected ourselves, then without a doubt we also reduce the nurturing care we lavish on the bacteria.[7]

Spiritual thoughts make all the difference
Much more could be done than anything put forward against bacteria nowadays by materialistic science, hugely more could be contributed to the future of humanity if only one were able to put forward ideas which might turn people away from materialism and encourage them towards an active love for the spirit. It is essential during this century for knowledge

to be propagated about the spiritual world and about how that world is so very relevant for our physical life, how it is profoundly significant for the physical world because we do indeed spend the time between going to sleep and waking up in that world whence we continue to exercise influence over our physical body.[8]

The force of healing has to work through community

We shall have to get used to the idea that something that can be seen as the healing force of spiritual science must begin to work through the human community. What would be the point if, upon going to sleep, an isolated individual here and there were to enter into the spiritual world with positive thoughts about that world if he were surrounded on all sides by others who—with their materialistic thoughts and feelings and fears, which are always linked with materialism—persisted in caring for and nurturing the world of the bacteria.[9]

Parasitic entities, creatures of Ahriman

What actually is this world of the bacteria? This question brings us to a subject which is closely linked with the life of human beings. Out there in nature we see the air filled with birds of all kinds, we see the water filled with fish, we see the animals bestirring themselves on the face of the earth. All these creatures in outer nature, perceived by us with our senses, are beings about which we rightly say that whatever form they take, even if from time to time they interfere in a damaging way with natural processes, they are nonetheless creations of an evolving divine world. But when we come to entities which live and work inside other living beings, in plants, in animals or human beings, then we have to say, especially in the case of bacteria or similar entities living inside animal or specifically in human bodies, that these are certainly also created by spiritual beings, namely by Ahriman. The correct view to take concerning these entities which live in our world is that they are all linked with spiritual facts, namely with the relationships between the human being and Ahriman. As we know, these relationships between the human being and Ahriman are brought about by a materialistic mindset or by egoistic states of fear. So the correct way to view the situation in which parasitic entities are present in the world is to understand that wherever such parasitic entities are to be seen they are symptoms of Ahriman's interference in the world.[10]

Bacteria: the symptom, not the cause, of a disease

We are taking a very superficial view of the matter if we imagine that diseases are caused by all the flora—and also fauna, as we shall see—that appear in the intestine or anywhere else in the human organism. It is really terrible to start to examine the literature on pathology today; in every chapter you come across statements about the discovery that this bacterium is associated with this disease or that bacterium with that disease, and so forth. All of these facts are extremely interesting as far as the botany and zoology of the human intestines are concerned; but none of it has any significance for illness except possibly as a sign that allows us to recognize the disease, because when one or the other form of disease is present, the human organism can be said to offer one or the other interesting little animal or plant a substrate upon which it can develop. It does not mean anything more than this. The growth of microscopic fauna and flora has very little to do with the actual disease—only indirectly, if at all.[11]

Directing attention to the habitat, not the bacteria

The presence of these interesting creatures tells us only that the habitat suits them, nothing more. We need to focus on studying this habitat ... Of course it can happen that the bacterial invasion provokes a well-prepared habitat to succumb to disease processes of its own accord. In reality, however, current bacteriological studies have nothing to do with the study of disease.[12]

Too much sleep predisposes towards epidemic illnesses

We have noticed the occurrence of so-called epidemic illnesses which take hold of whole swathes of a population and therefore also have social implications. The customary materialistic sciences study these epidemics with reference to the human organism. But they know nothing about the immensely important role that is played in connection with epidemics and the predisposition towards them by the abnormal conduct of human beings in connection with waking up and going to sleep. There is something which takes place in the organism when a human being is asleep, something which, if there is too much of it, thoroughly predisposes a person towards the so-called epidemic diseases. Individuals who, through sleeping too much, bring about processes in their organism that should not be there, because sleep ought not to interrupt waking life for such long periods, have an altogether different predisposition towards epidemic illnesses, and they also enter into an epidemic in an entirely different way.

You can imagine the difficulty of explaining to people about the proper ratio between sleeping and waking. Nothing can be achieved by means of rules and regulations analogous to stipulations regarding, for example, not sending one's children to school if they have scarlet fever ... Of course it is important to ensure that those who need to are able to sleep for seven hours while those who do not need so much may sleep for shorter periods and so on. Nevertheless, matters that are so intimately bound up with the most personal aspects of human life do have very great social consequences.[13]

Fixing attention on the bacteria distracts us from the primary causes of disease

In recent times the tendency has become ever more pronounced to disregard the actual causes and to look at surface occurrences. A phenomenon related to this superficiality is the fact that whenever we begin to read or hear a description of any type of illness, current medicine or pathology almost always informs us about what has invaded the human organism, about what kind of bacterium provokes the illness in question. It is terribly easy, of course, to repudiate any objections to the idea of lower organisms invading the body for the simple reason that it is no longer necessary first to prove that these lower organisms are present. Since distinct forms of micro-organisms are indeed evident in different illnesses, the tendency to suggest a connection is quite understandable.

But even on a superficial level, this view gives rise to an error that actually completely distracts us from the main issue. If bacteria appear in numbers in a certain part of the body in the course of an illness, they naturally provoke symptoms, as do any foreign bodies in the organism. As a result of the presence of these bacteria, all kinds of inflammations appear. But if we then attribute everything to the activity of the bacteria, directing our attention only to what the bacteria are doing, we are distracted from the true cause of the disease, because any habitat that lower organisms find suitable for their own development within the human body is brought about by the primary causes. For once we need to pay attention to the domain of primary causes.[14]

Confusing cause with effect

If someone's knowledge obliges him to maintain that the primary cause of an illness involving bacteria is something more profound than those bacteria, this does not mean that he is denying the presence of the bacteria. It is altogether different to point out that the bacteria are present and that they arise due to the illness, rather than maintaining that the bacteria are the primary cause ...

Let us imagine looking at a landscape full of beautiful, well cared for cattle. I might then ask: 'Why are these particular living conditions present in this region?' And I might answer: 'These conditions are brought about by these beautiful cattle.' In saying this I would be declaring that the living conditions in the region result from the arrival of the cattle which have multiplied here.

But I would not say such a thing, would I? I would look for

the primary causes, the diligence and understanding of the country folk, and this would explain why these beautiful cattle are flourishing on this land. I would be making a superficial statement if I were to say only: 'It is nice here, it's a good place to live because these beautiful cattle have arrived here.'[15]

Primary and secondary causes

If we survey modern allopathic medicine, we invariably find that it tends to evaluate patients with a view to the concomitant phenomena described by the bacterial theory of infection. This diverts our attention to a secondary issue. As a mere aid to recognition, the natural history of bacteria would be extremely useful. We can indeed learn a lot from the type of bacterium that is present, because a certain type always appears under the influence of a very specific primary cause. There is always plenty of opportunity to see this connection.

But there is a tendency to mistake a secondary factor for the primary cause, as when, for example, we look at the extent to which the bacteria affect human organs instead of the extent to which the human organism can become a habitat for bacteria. Such a tendency appears not only in allopathic medical theories concerning bacteria, but also in that whole way of thinking. Consequently, this tendency causes damage that I need not elucidate, since many of you have noticed it yourselves.[16]

Bacteria are everywhere, but they thrive where there is a source of infection

We have a constant interchange of life-giving air when we breathe in and death-bringing air when we breathe out.

Living and dying are constantly within us. And you will agree that it is very interesting to see how this living and dying becomes a part of the human being. To help you understand this, let me draw your attention to the fact that minute living creatures, bacteria, are present everywhere in nature. Countless such living creatures are flying all around us as we walk along surrounded by the air.

A muscle taken from an animal is full of countless tiny living creatures. And these tiny living creatures have the characteristic of multiplying hugely. One alone will scarcely have arrived before there are millions, especially of those that are smallest; they multiply hugely. The so-called infectious diseases rest on this. Not that these tiny living creatures cause the disease; but as soon as something in us falls sick these tiny living creatures thrive. Like plants growing on manure, these minute living creatures thrive within us in organs that are sick. They like being there. Anyone claiming that diseases come from the tiny living creatures, saying, perhaps, that influenza comes from the flu bacterium, might just as well maintain that the rain comes from the frogs he can hear croaking. Of course the frogs croak when it rains since being in the water they sense the rain's arrival and the stimulus it brings. The frogs do not bring the rain just as the bacteria do not bring influenza. But they are present where flu is present just as the frogs inexplicably appear when the rain comes.

So on the one hand we should not say that researching bacteria is pointless. They do after all show that human beings are susceptible to disease, just as the frogs croak when it rains. We should not throw the baby out with the bathwater by saying that researching bacteria is unnecessary. But on the other hand we ought to know that the bacteria do not cause the illness. It will never be correct to declare that there are bacteria for cholera and bacteria for influenza and so on. To do this is pure laziness because we cannot be bothered to investigate the true causes of disease.[17]

The cholera bacterium can live only in the human intestine

When you remove such bacteria, such minute living creatures, from their surroundings they can no longer stay alive. For example you cannot remove a cholera bacterium from the human intestine and let it live just anywhere. This is not possible. It can live only in human intestines or in the intestines of rats and similar animals. These minute creatures always need a specific environment in order to live.

Why is this so? That these tiny living creatures have a specific environment is a very important fact. When the cholera bacterium, let's say, is inside the human intestine it is less affected by the force of gravity than when it has been removed. The earth's gravity ruins the cholera bacterium when it is outside its element ...

So the cholera bacterium has to live inside the intestine of the human being. All bacteria have to live where they are protected from the earth. But what does it mean to be protected from the earth? It means that something other than the earth can have an effect on them. The fact is that the moon has an effect on all these living creatures. It may seem strange that the moonlight, which shines upon the earth now in one way and now in another, should have an effect on all these living creatures. But the fact is that it does. These living creatures have to be protected from the earth so that they can give themselves up to the cosmos, to the great universe, and chiefly to the influence of the moon.[18]

Too much protein increases susceptibility to infectious diseases

Human as well as animal bodies need not only the protein-generating forces they carry within themselves, for every living body does generate protein, but also the protein generated quite independently by plants. The human body does of course also absorb animal protein. But regarding this protein science has recently perpetrated a rather foolish mistake. About 20 years ago we were taught that the human body needed to take in at least 120 grams of protein every day in order to remain healthy. So the rules of nutrition everywhere stipulated which foods ought to be eaten in order to ensure the necessary intake of protein. Yes, people believed 120 grams to be necessary.

Today, science has backtracked very thoroughly about this. It is now known that eating too much protein not only does not serve to bring about good health but does in fact directly make us ill because most of the protein taken into the human intestine putrefies there. So eating 120 grams of protein every day causes the intestine to be filled with something like bad eggs, and this pollutes the content of the intestine dreadfully as poisons are exuded which are then absorbed by the body. There they bring about what in later life comes to be recognized as arteriosclerosis—for most arteriosclerosis is caused by eating too much protein—and they also make us very susceptible to all kinds of disease. The less protein we eat—while always remembering that a certain amount is necessary—the greater is our resistance to infectious disease. Those who eat large amounts of protein succumb more easily to infectious diseases such as diphtheria and smallpox than do those who eat less.

It is rather strange that science should now be telling us that 20 to 50 grams of protein are needed, and not 120 grams, that this smaller amount is sufficient for our daily needs. What a rapid turnaround in two decades! So you see how sceptical we should be when we are told that such-and-such has been scientifically proven. Looking for information about something, we might happen to read in a 20-year-old encyclopaedia that we need to eat 120 grams of protein. And then in a later edition we discover that more than 20 to 50 grams will make us ill.[*] That's how things are with regard to scientific facts. What is true or false varies with the edition of the encyclopaedia we happen to be consulting.[19]

Pain inflicted on animals in the past is re-embodied as parasitic causes of disease

Spiritual research tells us that all pain and all death inflicted by human beings on animals returns and rises up again, not through reincarnation but because pain and suffering have been inflicted on the animals. The animals on which pain has been inflicted do not come alive again in the same form, but the pain they have felt does return. It returns in a way that balances out the pain suffered by the animals, so that to every

---

[*] The recommendation nowadays is approximately 1 g per 1 kg of body weight per day. (Ed.)

pain its opposite feeling is added. This pain, this suffering, this death are seeds sown by human beings. They return and cause the opposite feeling to be added to every pain in the future.

Here is a concrete example. When the earth comes to be replaced by Jupiter,[*] the animals will no longer appear in their present form, but their pain and suffering will reawaken the powers which were sensitive to pain. They will live in human beings as parasitic creatures. And through what those people feel and sense, the balance will be created for the pain. This is the spiritual truth of the matter told objectively; it is the unvarnished truth even though today it makes us feel uncomfortable. Human beings will suffer this, and the animals will experience the balancing out of their pain in a feeling of comfort. This is indeed already happening slowly and gradually even in the present course of the earth's existence, strange though this may sound. Why are human beings tortured by entities which are neither animals nor plants but something in between, entities which enjoy making human beings suffer, namely bacteria and similar creatures? Human beings have brought this destiny upon themselves in earlier incarnations by inflicting suffering and death on the animals. Even if a creature does not appear again in the same form, nonetheless it feels the balancing out of pain and suffering which the human beings then have to experience. So whatever takes place by way of suffering and pain is not without consequences. There can be no suffering, no pain and no

---

[*] Steiner's term for a future incarnation of the earth.

death which does not bring into being something which will rise up again later.[20]

The trash of civilization as germs of disease

As you walk along a city street where your soul is presented with all kinds of hideous things in shop windows and on advertising displays, this has a gruesome effect on you. Materialistic science has no idea how many sources of disease lurk in these hideous things. Bacteria are thought to be the only causes of disease, so people do not realize how both bad and good health are drawn into the body via the soul. Those, however, who have gained an understanding of spiritual science will realize what can come into being when one absorbs one kind of picture or another as an internal image.[21]

In childhood illnesses such as scarlet fever and measles the individuality is battling with the inherited physical body

Legs are only meaningful when the earth's forces of gravity pass through them, when they are brought into the sphere of earthly gravity. It is only on the earth that legs, as well as arms and hands, have a purpose, which means that one whole part of our organization, in the way it has developed, is only meaningful when we are human beings living on the earth. What we are as human beings on the earth has no meaning as far as the cosmos is concerned. So when we arrive on the earth as beings of spirit and soul we have the wish to build up an entirely different organization. We want to set up a boundary within which we can create various configurations, but we do not yet want a body that means nothing to the cosmos. It is given to us as a model and we set up our second body to fit in with this model.

In the first period of our life on earth there is therefore a constant struggle between what has come to us from our previous life on earth and what we are presented with out of the stream of heredity. There is conflict between these two, and the illnesses of childhood are an expression of this strife. Just consider how intimately bound up our whole inner existence of soul and spirit is with our physical body during early childhood. When the second dentition begins you can see how the second tooth pushes out the first, how they engage in battle with one another; and the second human being as a whole engages with the first in the same way. In the second human being, however, the super-earthly being is present while in the first there is only an alien earthly model. These two engage with one another. And if you observe this mutual engagement correctly you will notice how the inner part, which was present as a being of spirit and soul during the existence prior to birth, gains the upper hand for a while on account of battling especially strongly against the physical through being forced to conform too strongly with the model. And you will notice that it damages the model as it clashes with it, saying: 'I want to create this particular form out of you.' This battle expresses itself in scarlet fever. But if the inner human being is so delicate that it keeps retreating although it wants to form the assimilated substances more in accordance with its own nature, its fight with the model then takes the form of measles. This is a struggle that expresses itself in the illnesses of childhood.[22]

In medicine, nothing can be comprehended with the intellect

It is dreadful that people today want to understand everything with their intellect. In medicine, nothing at all can be grasped by the intellect. At best one might be able to comprehend diseases suffered by the minerals, but it is of course not up to us to cure these. Everything in the field of medicine must be grasped through direct perception, so the faculty of direct perception must be developed for this purpose.[23]

Protection against infection: Approach infected persons without fear

The danger of becoming infected is exceptionally high in the case of smallpox. But we should not be so incautious as to think only of physical contagion as being the cause of becoming infected. In the case of smallpox specifically, psychological tendencies are especially strongly involved. Proof of this may be seen in the fact that one can very well gain protection by distancing oneself in the right way. I can vouch for this personally, for when I was 22 years old—never mind the circumstances—I was tutoring a pupil whose mother, who had smallpox, lay in the same room, separated from us only by a screen. I did nothing about this and continued with the lessons until the mother had recovered. Actually I rather enjoyed it because I wanted to see whether one could protect oneself by regarding the person with smallpox entirely objectively, like a stone or a bush towards which one has neither feelings of fear nor any other kind of psychological emotion but which one simply accepts as an objective fact. And I found that one can indeed protect oneself in high measure against contracting the disease. It stands to reason, therefore, that psychological factors can also play a large part in causing one to become infected.

Altogether, I have never been afraid of putting myself in a situation which might involve becoming infected, and I have never been infected nor have I contracted an infectious illness. On account of this I have also been able to confirm that a strong awareness of an illness can, in itself, become the cause of catching it through the intervention of the astral body.[24]

Do not be fanatical in the matter of vaccination

And what about vaccination against smallpox? This is a specific case. If one vaccinates someone but also educates that person in an anthroposophical way, no damage will be done. Such vaccination is only damaging to someone who grows up thinking chiefly materialistic thoughts. In this case, vaccination becomes a kind of ahrimanic force, so that the individual cannot rise above a certain degree of materialistic feelings. The cause for concern regarding the smallpox vaccination is that the individual becomes as it were inwardly clothed with a phantom. That person has a phantom which prevents him from extricating his soul elements from his physical organism as is the case in normal consciousness. Such a person become constitutionally materialistic and can no longer rise to spiritual things.

This is the risk with regard to vaccination. Of course statistics are always put forward in such situations, but it is questionable whether much store can be set by statistics in these matters. In the case of smallpox vaccination it is the soul element that is important. And of course the belief that vaccination will help plays a large role here. If one could put something else in the place of this belief—if one can educate human beings in ways which befit their nature so that they can be affected by something other than the matter of vaccination and can instead come closer once more to the spiritual element—then it would be quite possible to work against the unconscious thought: 'Here comes a smallpox epidemic!' If it were possible instead to be completely aware: 'Here comes something spiritual, something spiritual which is undesirable against which I must remain firm'—then this would be just as effective in making people strong in opposition to such influences.

A question from the audience: 'Where I live, for example, the effect of education and so on is very difficult, so what should I do about it?'

Well, in such situations you have to vaccinate. There's nothing for it. Not for medical reasons but on general anthroposophical grounds I would emphatically not recommend any fanatical opposition to vaccination. We are not aiming to put up a fanatical opposition to these things; what we want to do is change things in an overall way by means of insight. With any physicians who are friends of mine I have always made known my opposition to acting fanatically, for example in the case of Dr Asch who absolutely insisted on not vaccinating. I have always been against this attitude. If one doctor doesn't vaccinate, well then, another will. It is entirely absurd to act fanatically in isolation.[25]

*Distinguishing between primary causes and
infection, with tuberculosis as an example*

Contagion is still a valid concept here, however, because
people who are gravely ill with tuberculosis do affect their
fellow human beings, and exposure to a tubercular patient's
environment can indeed make it possible for what is otherwise a mere effect to once again become a cause. I always
attempt to use an analogy or comparison to clarify this
relationship between the primary genesis of a disease and
contagion. Let us assume I meet a friend in the street whose
personal relationships normally do not concern me. This
friend is sad, and with good reason, because one of his
friends has died. I have no direct connection to the deceased
person, but upon meeting my friend and hearing about his
grief I begin to feel sad with him. His sadness, however, is
due to a direct cause, while mine is due to contagion. But it
remains true that only the relationship between myself and
my friend supplies the necessary prerequisite for this contagion.

In this way, concepts of primary occurrence and contagion
are both fully justified, especially with regard to tuberculosis.
These concepts, however, really need to be applied ration-
ally. Tuberculosis sanatoriums are sometimes actual breeding grounds for tuberculosis. If tubercular patients have to be
crammed together in sanatoriums, then at least these build-
ings should be torn down periodically and replaced with new
ones whenever possible. After a certain length of time,
tuberculosis sanatoriums always ought to be replaced. The
strange thing about it is that tubercular patients themselves
have the greatest predisposition to infection, which means

that otherwise curable patients with the illness may become worse if they are in the proximity of those who are more seriously ill.[26]

Sunlight destroys tubercular bacteria

I don't know whether many of you experienced how truly awful it was some time ago when those ridiculous prohibitions against spitting in public came into effect everywhere in the attempt to combat tuberculosis. Such prohibitions are ridiculous for the simple reason that, as everyone should know, even ordinary sunlight kills tubercle bacteria in a very short time. If you examine sputum after a very short time, there are no more tubercle bacteria in it. Sunlight kills them immediately. Even if the supposition of ordinary medicine were correct, prohibiting spitting would still be highly ridiculous. At most such prohibitions make sense in terms of ordinary cleanliness, but not in terms of public hygiene in the broadest sense.

If we once again begin to assess the facts correctly, this example is very significant because it reminds us that the bacterium belonging to the fauna or flora of tuberculosis cannot survive in sunlight. The bacterium cannot survive there; it is not adapted to sunlight. But where can it survive? In the interior of the human body. And why can it survive precisely there? (Not that it does the actual damage, but we do have to look at what is active in the diseased body.) Here we encounter a situation we have tended to disregard. We are constantly surrounded by light, and light—as you probably recall from studying science—is extremely significant in the development of non-human organisms and especially for all the flora outside the human being. We are surrounded by this light. But something very significant happens to this light, which is purely etheric, at the boundary between ourselves and the outer world—it is, and must be, transformed.

You see, just as the process of becoming plantlike is arrested by human beings, interrupted and counteracted by the formation of carbon dioxide, what is active in the light is also broken off. Thus, if we look for light within the human being, it must be different, a metamorphosis of light. As soon as we cross the boundary into the interior of the human being, we find metamorphosed light. This means that we human beings not only transform ordinary, tangible natural processes within ourselves, we also transform intangibles. We transform light; we turn it into something else. If judged correctly, the fact that the tubercle bacterium does well within the human being but immediately perishes in the presence of sunlight is simply evidence that this bacterium is in its element in the product of the transformation of light that appears inside the human being. Therefore, if the bacterium thrives too well there, something must be wrong with this transformed light.

Taking this finding as your starting point, you can realize that one of the causes of tuberculosis must be the fact that within the human being (who would otherwise not take in an excess of ever-present tubercle bacteria) something that should not happen is happening to this transformed light, this metamorphosis of light. Tubercle bacteria are always present, although not in sufficient quantities, but they are superabundant in a person who contracts tuberculosis. Tubercle bacteria would not be present to such an extent if something abnormal were not taking place with regard to the process of transforming sunlight.

I can present these ideas only as points of view, of course, but you will be overwhelmed by the empirical confirmation that you will encounter. If a sufficient number of dissertations and treatises are written on this subject, it will not be difficult to discover that what happens when an individual becomes a suitable breeding ground for tubercle bacteria is due either to that person's reduced ability to take in sunlight or to a lifestyle that does not allow him or her to get enough sunlight, so that the appropriate balance does not exist between the sunlight entering the person and the light-metamorphosing process. As a result, the person in question has to draw down reserves of internal metamorphosed light.[27]

The fact of infection plays no part in the healing process
You see, those who want to learn about syphilis as an outer phenomenon, for example, will certainly be concerned with finding out to what extent contagion or at least some semblance of contagion is necessary in each case in order for syphilis to appear. Continuing in this vein eventually severs pathology from therapy. Pardon me if I use a somewhat crude comparison, but contagion is no more important in syphilis than the fact that in order to get a lump on the head the person in question must be hit by a stone or something else that delivers the blow. If this does not happen, no lump will develop. This is true enough, but enumerating the details does not result in a description that is productive for the healing process. The social significance of bricks or the like

falling on someone's head may be great, but with regard to studying the organism in order to arrive at a successful treatment, it does not have the slightest significance. We must study the human organism by looking for things that can play a role in therapy.[28]

2. KARMA AND EPIDEMICS

Susceptibility to epidemics through karma

What is present in the ether body in one life will come to expression in the physical body in the next life. A bad habit in a previous life leads to an illness in the next; and of course a good habit becomes the cause of good health. A specific passion will bring us a specific illness in our next life. It could be possible to see how a person's disposition towards infectious diseases comes about in this way. We know well how one person can visit anyone and go to all places where epidemics or infectious diseases are prevalent without being in any danger of contracting these diseases. Yet someone else picks every disease up off the street, as it were, and immediately becomes infected. Someone who is an initiate knows very well that a predisposition towards infectious diseases is the result of the former life in which the individual was very egoistically acquisitive and always strove to amass riches in a selfish way. A person wanting to grow rich in one life is causing himself damage in his next incarnation. This egoistic urge to gather possessions and riches is a characteristic of the ether body which in the next life lays down a disposition for contracting infectious diseases.[29]

The causes of disease and the karma of a nation

In seeking to gain information about health and sickness one must take into consideration that many factors all work together. The causes of disease do not necessarily lie in one's individual karma. In matters of disease there is also such a thing as the karma of a nation.[30]

Predispositions for disease may be attributed to specific characteristics in one's previous life

What develops in the ether body penetrates into the physical body in the next life. So not only do good inclinations and characteristics and efficient habits have the effect of making the physical body healthy in the next life, but also inefficient characteristics, bad habits and depraved inclinations come to expression in a sick organism. This should not be taken to mean that a specific disease stems from a specific characteristic but that certain predispositions to disease always lead back to specific characteristics and traits of temperament in a former life. So someone who has lived a life with depraved characteristics will have in his present life an organism that is more prone to physical illnesses than may be the case with another person. An individual who was equipped with healthy characteristics and a sound temperament will be reborn in a body that can be exposed to every kind of epidemic without becoming infected, and vice versa.

So you see how happenings in the world are linked in a complicated manner with the law of cause and effect.[31]

Genuine and illusory causes of illness

People often maintain that in days gone by the crassest superstitions were believed. Truly startling examples are cited of the methods used to heal one disease or another. And the use of certain terms is thought especially reprehensible, terms which in the past meant something that has long since been forgotten but which are nevertheless still used today although they are no longer understood. So now we say indignantly: 'There were times when every illness was ascribed either to God or to the devil!' But this is not as inappropriate as it seems; the fact of the matter is that we no longer know about the whole complex of views contained in the concepts of 'God' or 'the devil'. Perhaps an example will clarify this.

Suppose one person says to another: 'I've just been in a room which was full of flies; but someone told me that this was perfectly natural, and I believe him, since the room was very dirty, which makes it possible for the flies to survive there. It's easy to accept that the dirt is assumed to be the reason for the presence of the flies, and I believe him when he says that the flies will disappear when the room is thoroughly cleaned.'

But then someone else comes along and puts forward another reason for the presence of the flies, and that is that the room has long been inhabited by an exceedingly idle housewife. I'm sure you can see how utterly superstitious this is, as though idleness were some kind of personage who only needed to wave a hand for the flies to come in! The more reasonable of the two explanations is definitely that the presence of so much dirt is what has attracted the flies!

In another context this is very much like declaring that someone has fallen ill because he has been given an infection by some kind of bacterium and he will be well again when the bacteria have been driven out. So why on earth do some people go on about there being a more deep-seated spiritual reason! All you need to do is chase away the bacteria! It is no more superstitious to talk about the spiritual cause of an illness, while recognizing all the other causes, than it is to explain the presence of the flies being caused by an exceed-ingly idle housewife. There is no need to have an argument about getting rid of the flies by cleaning up.

The point is not to argue with one another but to learn to understand one another and listen carefully to what each has to say. This must be thoroughly taken into account when someone quite rightly talks of the more obvious direct causes of an illness as well as of those that are more distant. An objective anthroposophist will not insist that idleness only needs to wave her hand in order to invite the flies to enter the room. He will know perfectly well that other, physical cir-cumstances must also be taken into consideration. But at the same time he knows that everything which finds expression in the physical world also has a spiritual background and that in order to heal humanity this spiritual background must be taken into consideration as well.

Those who wish to take part in the argument need to be reminded that the spiritual causes must not always be given the same interpretation and cannot necessarily be counter-acted in the same way as the ordinary physical causes. And one should also not think that taking a stand against the spiritual causes exempts us from pressing forward against the physical causes. If one were to act in this way one could allow the room to remain dirty while only doing battle with the idleness of the housewife.[32]

Thorough investigation of an illness must include a consideration of karma

In their considerations about an illness, people today are very much inclined to consider only the most obvious causes. A

basic tenor of today's world view is to follow the most convenient route. The most convenient method in respect of
what causes an illness is to look only at the most obvious
causes—and those most inclined to do this are indeed often
the patients themselves ... But those who endeavour to study
karma in its most manifold effects will always extend their
view beyond what takes place in the present time in order to
include events that lie in the far distant past. They will above
all reach the conviction that a thorough understanding of the
facts of a case concerning a human being can only be gained
by opening up one's view to include the happenings of long
ago. This is especially the case where sicknesses are concerned.[33]

*How does a weak sense of self in an earlier incarnation
influence the likelihood of succumbing to an epidemic?*
Let us assume that in his previous life an individual func-
tioned with a sense of his own 'I' which was far too weak, a
sense of his 'I' which gave in far too readily to the outside
world so that the effect was one of dependency and loss of self
to an extent that is no longer appropriate in the present cycle
of human evolution. His lack of a sense of self caused him to
act in a certain way in an incarnation. In the period of
kamaloca he had before him the actions which flowed from
that lack of a feeling of self. The resulting tendency which
arises in him makes him say: I must develop forces within me
that increase my sense of self; in a future incarnation I must
create an opportunity to work against the resistance put up by
my body, against the forces which come to meet me from my
physical body, from my ether and astral bodies, so that my

sense of self is strengthened. I must develop a body which shows me the consequences of having a weak sense of self.

The individual will not be fully aware of what then takes place in the coming life, for it will have its effect more or less in a subconscious realm. He will strive towards having an incarnation in which his sense of self is confronted with the most robust resistance so that it has to exert itself to the utmost. He will be magnetically attracted to regions and opportunities that place stronger obstacles in his path and where his sense of self is forced to live to the full in opposition to the organization of the three bodies. Strange though this may seem to you, individuals who are burdened with a karma of entering into life in the way I have described will search out opportunities to be born in a place where they will be exposed, for example, to a cholera epidemic. This is what will give them the opportunity to practise the kind of resistance I have been describing. What the sick individual will have to undergo inwardly in opposing his three bodies can then lead in his next incarnation to a considerable enhancement of his sense of self.[34]

How does a strong sense of self in an earlier incarnation influence the likelihood of succumbing to an epidemic?
Let us now take another striking example, namely the opposite case, to help you understand what all this is about. During his time in kamaloca an individual sees that he performed a number of actions under the influence of a sense of self that was too powerful. He realizes that he must restrain his sense of self, that he must subdue it somewhat. He must now seek out opportunities in his next incarnation in which his three bodies

in the new incarnation do not confront him with any obstacles so that—however hard he might try—there will be no limitations. The conditions for this will be presented when he is attracted to a situation in which he will encounter malaria.

Here we have a case of an illness brought about by karma. And this also explains how an individual is led, by an intelligence higher than that available to his normal consciousness, towards opportunities for developing himself further during the course of his karma. If you bear in mind what we have been discussing you will find it easy to understand the significance of the epidemic nature of illnesses. There are many possible examples all of which would show how an individual, through experiences in kamaloca, comes to seek out opportunities for contracting one illness or another so that by overcoming it, and by gaining more forces of self-healing, he can be led upward along the path of life.[35]

Is it permissible to impede karmic compensation by means of preventive measures against epidemics?
How is it that as human beings on earth we must ... endeavour to correct the harmful influences of the Ancient Moon forces? As humans on earth we will surely sense that we should not wish for volcanic eruptions and earthquakes and that we are not permitted to destroy our organs ourselves in order to support the beneficial working of the spiritual powers. But we should be able to say to ourselves with some justification: When an epidemic breaks out somewhere, this is because it will bring something into being which we are seeking so that a balancing out may occur. And we may assume that we are driven into certain situations so as to

experience some specific damage, for in overcoming that damage we shall overcome ourselves in a way that will take us further in our quest for greater perfection.

But what is the situation with regard to hygienic and sanitary measures? Might not someone say: 'Aha, so epidemics are a good thing! Therefore it must be wrong to institute all kinds of health-promoting arrangements in order to prevent such influences from playing their part?' ...

We shall see that this is not the case, although only under certain circumstances. We are now ready in our next discussion to understand situations in which beneficial influences actually inflict damage on an organ in order on the one hand to prevent us from falling victim to maya, but on the other hand to make us aware of the effects we bring about when we sidestep such beneficial influences by instituting sanitary and hygienic measures against diseases.[36]

Measures that counter the karmic effects of epidemics

There have been times when humanity was not capable of instituting measures to counteract epidemics. Those were the days when the overall wise plan for the world intended epidemics to work in a way that would give human souls the opportunity to counterbalance what had come about through ahrimanic influence and also through certain earlier luciferic influences. Nowadays different preconditions are being introduced, and this is once again taking place under the auspices of certain broader karmic laws. So obviously we should not consider these questions in a superficial way.

How does this agree with our statement that if an individual seeks an opportunity to become infected during an epidemic this is a necessary way of countering a cause stemming from a previous incarnation? Do we, then, have the right to institute hygienic and other measures against this?

This is a profound question, and we shall have to gather the right information before replying to it. We must understand that where the luciferic and the ahrimanic principles work either in concert or in opposition to one another—whether simultaneously or over longer periods of time—certain complications arise in human life. These complications occur in all kinds of situations and in numerous ways so that no two cases will be the same. However, in studying human life we shall be able to find our way as follows. In endeavouring to discover how Lucifer and Ahriman work together in a specific case we shall always find a thread of continuity which clarifies the connection. We must, however, distinguish clearly between what is internal and what is external. Nowadays we have to differentiate between what lives in the intellectual soul and what lives in the ether body as an effect of the intellectual soul. We must observe the process by means of which karma is accomplished, but we must at the same time understand that we can also work on the inner being by means of appropriate karmic influences in a way that will enable the inner being to prepare for a different karmic compensation in the future.[37]

Creating a spiritual counterbalance when institutionalized health measures interfere with karmic effects

Let us suppose that out of a lack of charity towards humanity quite a number of individuals were tempted to absorb infectious substances in order to succumb to an epidemic. And let us in addition suppose that we were in a position to do something against the epidemic. In such a case we would protect the external physical body from giving expression to a lack of charity but we would not have removed the inner tendency towards such lack of charity. But then let us imagine that in removing the organic basis for a lack of charity we also commit ourselves to removing the tendency towards a lack of charity in the soul. The organic basis for a lack of charity is killed in the external bodily sense by vaccination against smallpox. The following is made clear by this, as has been researched by spiritual science: Smallpox developed during a cultural period when there was a general tendency towards a greater degree of egoism, of uncharitableness ...

This helps us to understand how vaccination came into being in our age. But we can also understand that a kind of aversion against vaccination has also arisen among the best minds of our period. This corresponds with something internal; it is the external expression of something internal. So if on the one hand we destroy the physical organization we could say that we also have the duty, as a countermeasure, to transform that individual's materialistic character by means of a suitable spiritual education. This would constitute the necessary countermeasure without which we would have performed only half the task. We would merely have succeeded in bringing about the necessity for the individual in question to produce the countermeasure himself in a subsequent incarnation ... In destroying the susceptibility to smallpox we have taken only the external aspect of the karmic effect into account. If we institute health measures on the one hand we must feel it our duty on the other hand to give those whose physical organization we have transformed something for their soul. Vaccination will do no damage to people so long as they subsequently receive a spiritually oriented education.[38]

Health measures called for by the great laws of human karma

This brings us to an important law in human evolution which results in there always being a balance between an external and an internal aspect so that when paying attention to the one we must not leave the other out of account. This gives us a glimpse of a very important inter-dependency without even having arrived yet at our discussion of the question: 'What is the relationship between health and karma?' ...

Let us suppose that by instituting health measures of some kind we render impossible certain causes, certain circumstances needed by an individual in connection with his karma. Let us imagine that we succeed in combating certain specific agents of disease. We have already shown that the taking of such measures does not lie within the choice of humanity. We have seen that in a certain period the tendency towards cleanliness, for example, is felt simply because it had disappeared in the intervening period and has now in a new period become necessary once again. We can glean from this that our adoption of one measure or another at a particular moment in history is governed by the great laws of human karma.[39]

The connection between physical well-being and psychological wretchedness

Consider a situation in which a number of individuals feel impelled by their karmic entanglements to seek out certain influences which would provide a balancing-out of karma for them. Health measures, however, have meanwhile done away with those influences or circumstances, so the individuals concerned cannot find them. Yet this does not free them from their need for a specific karmic effect, so they are obliged to seek out others instead. Human beings cannot escape their karma. Such measures do not free them from seeking what in other circumstances they would have sought...

It is a fact that a good number of external influences and causes are being removed which would otherwise have been sought as a means of balancing-out certain karmic matters with which humanity burdened itself in former times. All we do by instituting such measures is to remove the likelihood of falling prey to external influences. We merely make people's external life more congenial or more healthy. The only achievement has been to oblige people who would have found the karmic compensation they needed through a specific illness to look for this compensation by other means. The souls who have been saved by these measures in respect of their health are now condemned to look to other means for the compensatory karma they require ...

Having been granted greater physical comfort through enjoying better health their physical life has been made easier. But their soul is influenced in the opposite way. In their soul they gradually come to experience an emptiness, a dissatisfaction, a sense of being unfulfilled. If external life were to continue growing ever more enjoyable and ever more healthy in accordance with the general idea of what our purely materialistic life could be like, such souls would increasingly lack a stimulus to work at their own development. Psychological wretchedness would constitute the parallel development.

This is already becoming evident to those who look at life more closely. It is unlikely that there has ever been an age in which people have lived such comfortable external lives while going about with such wretched, unfulfilled souls. These people hurry from one sensational event to the next; if their financial situation permits they travel from city to city in order to see the sights; or if they are obliged to remain in one city they rush from one entertainment to the next, evening after evening. Yet their soul life remains wretched in no longer knowing what to look for in the world which might yield some worthwhile content ... Souls suffer increasingly while external life grows ever more healthy.[40]

3. THE SPIRITUAL BACKGROUND OF EPIDEMICS

Bacteria: a consequence of ahrimanic hosts having been cast down upon the earth

The forces present in bacteria, and whatever bacteria do, are a consequence of the ahrimanic hosts of heaven having been cast down upon the earth, of the dragon having been conquered. Another consequence of that victory is that the ahrimanic-mephistophelian way of thinking has been spreading across the earth since the end of the seventies [of the nineteenth century]. We can therefore say that on the physical level diseases involving bacteria and equally also present-day intellectual materialism have their source in the realm of soul and spirit. In a higher sense the two things are most certainly comparable.[41]

Cosmic rhythms and epidemic diseases

For example, although rats carry certain epidemic diseases it cannot be said that a disease comes from the rats; they are merely the carriers which spread the disease. Similarly, in reality bacteria have nothing to do with all that goes to make up the disease as such. Just as events of spirit and soul lie behind the outer symptoms of history, so do cosmological events lie behind the manifestations of bodily states of health. It is the rhythmical course of cosmic events that is important. This is what we must study. We should ask what cosmic constellations surrounded us during the eighties [of the nineteenth century] when today's influenza appeared in its milder form. And in what cosmic constellations are we living at present? What is going on in the cosmic rhythm to cause the earlier form of influenza to appear again now more severely? Just as we have to discover the rhythms in the sequence of historical events, so must we look for a specific rhythm that lies behind the occurrence of certain epidemic diseases.[42]

Medical science must be founded on cosmological symptomatology

Do you believe that people will really begin to understand these things unless they condescend to look at a proper cosmology with the help of spiritual science? It was thought foolish—and in this form it is indeed foolish—when it was said: The tendency of humanity to make war is connected with sun-spot periods. But a point will always be reached when even a statement of this kind is no longer regarded as entirely foolish, namely when it is said that the occurrence of certain pathological impulses in connection with the life of the temperaments is linked with cosmological phenomena such as the rhythmically recurring sun-spot periods. And if these little chaps, these minute fellows—bacteria, rats—can really carry from one person to another something that has a cosmological connection, then this is a secondary matter although it can be easily proven. But it is not the main thing. Above all we must realize that we shall not be able to understand the main thing if we are unwilling to study the peripheral symptoms as well ...

It will also not be possible to make headway in matters of

public sanitation, hygiene and medicine if we do not study a cosmological, not a historical but a cosmological symptomatology. The fact is that whatever lives on the earth in the form of diseases is actually sent down from the heavens.[43]

4. PROTECTION DURING EPIDEMICS

Logical thinking as a protection during epidemics
Logical, clear thinking has a strengthening and health-promoting effect on the physical body, making it less susceptible to disease. Those who, like mathematicians, are accustomed to think in this way have less to fear when paying visits to cholera hospitals and such places ...

In this way confidence is established in all matters of outer and inner life. Strong individuals will listen only to their own inner voice while those who are weak are inclined to wait for advice and suggestions from others.[44]

The importance of sleep in relation to health and sickness
There is in our physical body something which is strengthened and invigorated by what our soul absorbs from the spiritual world while we are asleep, by what rays into it from out of the spiritual world. While we are asleep the sun of our 'I' and our astral body sets in respect of the life of our nerves and blood ... and begins to shine for the other organic processes in our body. So it is indeed really easy to understand that sleep is an important medicine and that unhealthy sleep is indeed one of the most influential causes of disease, especially with regard to certain inner processes of the body.[45]

Medieval fear of ghosts and modern fear of bacteria
As we know, human life changes with regard to some things, and yet certain fundamental nuances of life remain the same

over long periods of time. Thus there was a specific fear
during the Middle Ages, a fear that today is seen as darkest
superstition, namely the fear of ghosts, of all kinds of
elemental beings and sprites. For us today this is merely a
medieval superstition. Well, nowadays the object has
changed but the fear remains, for today it is not ghosts of
which we are afraid as was the case in the Middle Ages but so-
called bacteria and similar entities. Well, it could be said that
ghosts were relatively suitable as objects of fear, more so than
the entities nowadays known as bacteria and suchlike. All
that has changed is the fact that in those days people were
more spiritual and thus feared spiritual things such as the
elemental beings, whereas today we are more materialistic in
our outlook so that our ghosts must also be more physical.
This is perfectly in keeping with the age of materialism.[46]

Materialistic ideas carried over into sleep encourage bacteria

What I wanted to emphasize was the fact that spiritual
science does indeed show us that bacteria, for example, need
to be carefully tended in the human body if they are to
flourish properly. Human beings have to take care of them.
Of course anyone today will point out how foolish it would be
to take care of bacteria, to fatten them up and ensure their
multiplication in numbers. However, it is not a question of
having principles, whatever they may be, but of being able to
see the matter in its proper perspective. Thus knowledge
gained through spiritual science cannot deny that bacteria are
actively encouraged to flourish when, for example, an 'I' and
an astral body, which feed solely on materialistic ideas and

deny any spiritual perspectives, depart from the body during sleep without admitting that other forces from the spiritual world stream into the physical organs in their place and become greatly beneficial for the life of bacteria. If you really want to fatten up bacteria, there is no better method than to take crude materialistic ideas with you into sleep, thus calling up ahrimanic forces which pour into your organism and become nurses for the bacteria.[47]

The crucial importance of human community

In order to form a correct view of such a situation we must realize that as soon as we turn our attention to the life of the spirit it will be necessary to consider what is meant by the idea of human community. Collaboration within a human community is immensely more important in respect of the spiritual effects it brings about than it is in respect of the consequences that occur only on the physical plane. One might imagine that the best thing a person could do in order to prevent any bacteria from causing damage to his body would be to use the practice of going to sleep while thinking spiritual thoughts as a medicine. If this could be clinically proven, it might even be possible for the most hard-boiled materialists in the future to have the doctor prescribe spiritual ideas for them. Perhaps such a thing could even serve to promote spiritual life as such? But no, things are not as simple as that. In matters of the spirit it is the importance of community life that immediately gains enormous significance.

It has to be said that a single individual may not be helped at all by cultivating such spiritual ideas if those all around him foster bacteria through the use of materialistic ideas, for in this realm each individual fosters on behalf of all the others.

This is the important aspect about which we must be clear. As I have already said, one cannot sufficiently emphasize the fact that spiritual science as such cannot, on the basis of one individual alone, fruitfully fulfil the task it is supposed to fulfil for humanity. It is not enough for isolated individuals to take up spiritual science; spiritual science must wait patiently until it becomes a determining element of culture through entering into the hearts and souls of many individuals. Only then will we be shown what it can mean for human beings.[48]

Imaginations of fear strengthen the ahrimanic forces which are inimical to human beings

There is, though, something else that has an equally strong effect on the ahrimanic beings which can be observed in bacteria. The difference between ahrimanic beings and others is easily demonstrated, even externally. All around us we see nature with its creatures. Those which live outside in nature have been granted their life by the progressive, good and wise creators. But those which take up residence inside other organisms and flourish there are either of a luciferic or an ahrimanic type. All entities of a parasitic kind are either luciferic or ahrimanic in origin, and this makes it easy for us to distinguish them in nature.

There is, then, something else which is extraordinarily useful for these ahrimanic entities which live as parasites inside the human body. Imagine being surrounded by an epidemic. In such a situation one individual of course assists another so that the nature of human community and everything connected with it grows immensely strong, although karmic connections can bring it about that someone who might seem least likely to succumb to the epidemic does indeed succumb. Yet in general it is true—and we should not permit ourselves to be duped by appearances—that when one is surrounded by others who have succumbed or are dying, and when one has taken in these images before entering into sleep while having nothing but egoistic fear, then the imagination, which arises out of these images and then lives in the soul during sleep, becomes imbued with an egoistic fear which brings it about that harmful forces enter into the body.

It is imaginations of fear that provide the forces which nurture the ahrimanic enemies of human beings. If a magnanimous way of thinking begins to unfold, so that egoistic fear recedes, if loving assistance begins to work amongst the people so that they enter into sleep not with imaginations of fear but with all that is generated by the giving of loving assistance, then this causes damage to humanity's ahrimanic enemies.[49]

Much on earth depends on the spiritual life we take with us into sleep

There is no justification in maintaining that nothing connected with the life of the spirit need be a matter of concern to us while we live on the earth. In fact a great deal on earth depends upon the kind of spiritual life we take with us into sleep. What we take with us into sleep makes our soul either a good or a bad tool for all that rays into the organs of our body from the spiritual world. These tools are not derived from the soul life of our daytime consciousness but from the physical and chemical functions that take place underneath the threshold of consciousness. It is not a matter of how the nerves and the blood work but of how the circulation functions in the organs, the physical and chemical effects which are not those of plant or mineral life but rather of the spiritual forces which ray in from the spiritual world during sleep. That is why it is important to take into our life of sleep our spiritual knowledge and the frame of mind which emanates from that spiritual knowledge.[50]

The content of spiritual science makes us stronger

Once the world comes to realize the full significance of what spiritual science can accomplish here there will be a gradual decline in the importance attached to all those lovely—and I do not mean this ironically but entirely seriously—theories about infectious diseases and suchlike which are nowadays looked upon in a very one-sided way. Rather than examining the manner in which the bacteria enter into our organism, much more attention will be paid to the strength we have gained in our soul and our spirit with which to resist these infestations. There will be no external medicine which will lend our human nature the necessary strength. The medicine which will strengthen us will come from the spirit and the soul through the health-giving content of spiritual science.[51]

The effect of light on parasitic entities

Let us take the case of a patient whom we place in a situation where excessive amounts of light are at work so that he is surrounded by light which fills the air around him. We could express this by saying that the patient is in a region from which we have sent away the earthly influences and placed him instead under the influence of forces from outside the earth. Strong sunshine is filled with something which the earth no longer needs, which the earth repels. So the patient enters into the region where an influence comes from outside the earth. By placing the patient in air that is shone through by the sun we affect his rhythmic organism. We affect his rhythmic organism very strongly so that an irregular metabolism which is exposed to this light will regulate itself because of the strong influence that the rhythm has upon it.

This, then, explains how the treatment with light and air works for patients who are sent to a spa. Cures of this kind are especially recommended for patients who possess a very low resistance to parasitic invasions. There is no need to be an adherent of the theory of bacteria, for it is simply a matter of understanding that the presence of parasites indicates that there are more deep-seated reasons why the patients in question are prone to attracting and retaining bacteria. Bacteria are really never the actual cause of a disease but rather merely an indicator of the patient having the 'causes' within himself. Research into bacteria is important, of course, but its purpose is simply to find a knowledge basis for what is happening. The organic causes of the disease lie within the patient. And what works against these causes is something from the cosmos which approaches and surrounds the earth without being totally absorbed by it. It is a superabundance of something, a superabundance of sun, a superabundance of light and so on. This is what works effectively in these situations, something which is over and above what makes the earth sprout and germinate, something which makes it begin to sparkle and shine, something which contains more light than is needed merely for sprouting and germinating.[52]

5. PRESENT CAUSES OF FUTURE EPIDEMICS

Materialism leads to future epidemic diseases of the nervous system

Whatever we dump onto the astral plane today will appear on the physical plane tomorrow. What we sow on the astral plane we will reap on earth in future times. This indicates that we are today harvesting the fruits of the narrow-minded materialistic mentality sown on the astral plane by our predecessors.

So we may conclude how fundamentally important are spiritual truths. If science today were to accept the gifts of spiritual science, even if only as hypotheses, the whole world would change. Materialism has plunged human beings into depths which are so dark that an inconceivable effort will be required to extricate them once more. Humanity is falling under the influence of nervous diseases which are unfolding into very epidemics of psychological illness. Something which we here refer to as feelings and which is to be found on the astral plane is now returning to earth as a reality. Nervous disorders which exhaust human beings come from the astral plane.[53]

The karma of materialism: future epidemics of insanity

The materialism of science is in the first instance a consequence of materialism in religion; there would be no such thing if the religious life were not drenched in materialism.

Those who today are too lazy to enter into the religious realm in depth are the very ones who have generated the materialism of the sciences. This shattering of the nerves brought about by materialism is affecting whole swathes of the population, whole nations as well as individuals.

If the stream of spirituality fails to gain sufficient impetus and thus win over also those who are lazy and easy-going, then the karmic consequence, the nervous impairment, will increasingly influence humanity. Just as the Middle Ages saw epidemics of leprosy, so in future will the materialistic outlook generate serious nervous diseases, whole epidemics of insanity; and whole peoples will succumb.

Insight into this aspect of karmic law ought to bring it about that spiritual science is no longer a matter of dispute but something that can be a means of healing for the whole of humanity. The more humanity turns towards spirituality, the more will everything that has to do with diseases of the nervous system and of the soul be eliminated.[54]

The most harmful effect of materialism lies in the realm of the religious life

Karma is worked out not only in individuals but also in nations and indeed in humanity as a whole. If you have studied the history of spiritual life in Europe, you will know that materialism has been gaining ground over the last four hundred years or so. This materialism is least harmful in the sciences, for here any mistakes can easily be recognized and corrected. Its effects are far more damaging in practical life where everything is viewed from the angle of material interests. Never, however, would materialism have gained so much ground in practical life if human beings had not had a predisposition for it . . .

But materialism is at its most damaging in the realm of the religious life, that is, in the churches; the Church has for years been making its way towards materialism. Why is this? If you were to go back to the days of early Christianity you would never come across any claim that the creation of the world really took seven days to be completed as is so often presumed nowadays, and that the 'seventh day' should be imagined as a day during which someone sits down on a chair in order to rest after heavy physical exertion. Our materialistic age no longer has any knowledge about the reality of the 'seven days of creation'. It is now down to anthroposophy once again to enlighten humanity as to the true meaning of that ancient document known as Genesis.

The materialistic attitude in religion has penetrated most deeply into the life of the nations. It is an attitude which will dominate increasingly in the field of religion, so that here there will be less and less understanding of the spiritual as opposed to the physical, material element. You will surely admit that materialistic thoughts, feelings and will impulses have increasingly come to penetrate humanity's whole concept of life; and this will in the end put its stamp upon the health of future generations.[55]

Without spirituality, mental illnesses would attain epidemic proportions

An age which believed in nothing but physical matter would breed descendants with bodies in which there was no longer a proper centre, so that symptoms of neurasthenia and nervous disease would arise. This would spread more and more rapidly if materialism were to remain the chief world view in future. Someone who has spiritual insight can tell you exactly what would arise if materialism were not to be met with a counterweight in the shape of a firm view of the spirit. Mental illnesses would take on epidemic proportions, and even at birth children would show signs of nervousness and suffer from fits of trembling; and a further consequence of materialistic attitudes is a human race, such as we see around us even today, which lacks any powers of concentration.[56]

The law of karma is not about a blind faith in fate

So you see that when thinking more deeply about the law of karma one cannot regard the individual only as a solitary being but must also see him as he is situated within the law of karma as a part of the community as a whole. The law of karma is not something that can be comprehended by those who want to believe only in blind fatalism. To see the law of karma in this way is a complete and utter misunderstanding. Yet it is not unusual to come across people who do subscribe to this error. One such person might say: 'I know that I cannot do anything about this, for it is my karma and I have to live with it.' Or another says: 'There is a person who is suffering, but it is not up to me to help him because it is his karma, so he must live with it.' All such reactions amount to a completely nonsensical interpretation of the concept of karma![57]

Every kind of feeling brings about a change in the structure of the physical body

Something comes down from the higher worlds and takes possession of our physical body when we depart from it at night. Some forms of astral substantiality which created or participated in creating it, as well as the ether body, take hold of it once more. But they now find that it differs from how it was when they first provided us with it. We have been rummaging about in our physical body with our astral body and our 'I'; and the spiritual beings from the higher regions of the universe now find effects in it that are not compatible with their higher spirituality, effects that have arisen because of what we have been doing in it by means of our astrality and our 'I' during daytime ... It is impossible to have thoughts or feelings that do not have an effect right down into the physical body. No anatomist can prove this, but every kind of feeling we have brings about certain changes in the structure of the physical body, and this is what those higher beings find when they enter into us once again at night.[58]

Untruthfulness generates phantoms

Everything in the human soul that has to do with lying, with slander, with hypocrisy generates effects that are of special significance in what they do to the physical body. Seen from a materialistic point of view, lying, slander and hypocrisy are thought to have only those effects which can be observed externally. But this is not the case. Extremely subtle effects reach right down into the physical body although these cannot be detected even with microscopic instruments. So when the soul departs in sleep, these effects remain in the physical body and are found there by the spiritual beings. The experiences of soul which generate these effects are not only the coarser ones such as lying, slander and hypocrisy. Even little conventional lies, for example those made necessary today by social mores, are not without effect. Lying out of politeness or for the sake of good manners, and the whole range of insincerities and hypocrisy and minor aspersions—even only in thought—all this gets expressed in the effects on the physical body and is then found by the spirits when they descend.

And because all this is there within the physical body during the night something specific is brought about. Fragments of the substance of the beings descending into the body are torn off. Certain parts of those higher beings are tied off. The consequence of lying and hypocrisy and slander during the day is that at night certain beings are tied off and because of this they gain a kind of resemblance with the human physical body. They develop an independent existence in the spiritual world which surrounds us; they are beings of the class known as phantoms.

Phantoms are spiritual entities that express something in their external physiognomy through being in a way copies of the human form and its bodily members. Their materiality is so attenuated that they are invisible to our physical eyes, yet they do have what one must call a physical form. With clairvoyance one can see buzzing through the air pieces of human heads, human hands, whole bodies, and also of the insides of human bodies, the stomach, the heart, all these phantoms which have tied themselves off as a consequence of lying, hypocrisy and slander.[59]

Phantoms created through lying feed on bacteria
Phantoms which constantly buzz about in our spiritual environment are a proof to you that human life itself causes

entities to come into existence that affect human beings in ways that are by no means beneficial; they possess certain characteristics which are intelligent but have no moral feelings of responsibility. They keep their life on the go by putting obstacles in people's way, obstacles that are far greater than what we call bacteria. And something else happens as well. Important causes of illness can be found in such entities: having been created by human beings, these phantoms find very good opportunities for their existence in bacteria; one could even say that they feed on the bacteria. They would become quite desiccated in their spiritual nature if this food were not available. Yet on the other hand the bacteria are in a way also created by them ...

Human beings, then, create whole hosts of spiritual beings in the phantom class through lying, slander and hypocrisy.[60]

Inappropriate social regulations generate ghosts

The situation is similar in the case of the ether body from which the human being departs at night. The human ether body can only exist if it is permeated by higher beings, so when the astral body has departed those beings dip down into the ether body in its place. We must grasp this fully! If we do, we shall understand why it is that effects are brought about in our ether body by certain processes in our soul life, effects that remain during the night and cause entities to be tied off from the beings that descend into it. The soul processes that generate these entities are processes that come about when the life of the human community is regulated by what we might term unsuitable laws, inappropriate regulations. Many things brought about through inappropriate regulations, which the soul experiences as being wrong in social inter-course, lead to after-effects in the ether body during the night, effects which cause the entities we call ghosts to be tied off. This is the second type of entity among those which are created by the human being.[61]

Defective advice and prejudices generate demons

We must also take into consideration the fact that the reverse is also valid. That which departs during the night, the astral body, is organized in such a way that it is dependent on being encased in the nervous system ... So it, too, has to be cared for by higher worlds in that higher, guardian spirits have to unite with it. And from these spirits, too, something can be tied off as the result of specific soul processes which are caused by the effect on the human being of what we might term 'giving defective advice', forcing false advice on some-one, developing baseless prejudices, persuading others not through agreement but by inflicting convictions upon them which one holds fanatically oneself.

When the interpersonal relationship between individuals is like this, then an effect remains in the astral body during the night that ties off from the higher beings certain entities that belong to the class known as demons. They are generated as described when individuals interact with one another not with an attitude of tolerance which says, 'I will say what I think, but if the other person disagrees that is his affair' ... but rather with an attitude which says, 'If you don't share my opinion then you're a fool.' When one soul interacts with another in this way, demons are generated superabundantly.

Thus human life itself really does generate spiritual entities which then populate the spiritual world. All these entities—phantoms, ghosts and demons—conversely also affect human beings. When some prejudice or foolish fad appears on the scene on an epidemic scale, this is caused by the demons created by human beings, all of which impede the straight line of progress. Human beings are forever encircled by entities they themselves have created.[62]

Everything we think, feel and sense is at work all around us

We must realize that greater, more significant consequences arise from anything we think, feel and sense than from the firing of a shot. The latter may be bad, but it is only considered to be more dangerous because we are able to perceive it with our unsubtle senses, whereas we are incapable of observing those other consequences at all.[63]

NOTES

Given that this volume is made up of quotations from Rudolf Steiner's works, Steiner's words have been translated afresh from the latest and most accurate German editions in order to keep a consistent flow to the language, tone and terminology. 'GA' stands for *Gesamtausgabe* or Collected Works of Rudolf Steiner in the original German. Complete volumes translated into English are shown in 'Sources' on page 65.

1. Epidemics and Infection
1. Lecture in Berlin, 14 January 1909, GA 57.
2. Ibid.
3. Lecture in Hamburg, 20 May 1910, GA 120.
4. Lecture in Basel, 5 May 1914, GA 154.
5. Lecture in Mannheim, 5 January 1911, GA 127.
6. Lecture in Basel, 5 May 1914, GA 154.
7. Ibid.
8. Ibid.
9. Ibid.
10. Ibid.
11. Lecture in Dornach, 24 March 1920, GA 312.
12. Ibid.
13. Lecture in Dornach, 7 April 1920, GA 314.
14. Lecture in Dornach, 7 April 1920, GA 312.
15. Lecture in Dornach, 7 April 1920, GA 73a.
16. Lecture in Dornach, 9 April 1920, GA 312.
17. Lecture in Dornach, 23 December 1922, GA 348.
18. Ibid.
19. Lecture in Dornach, 23 January 1924, GA 352.
20. Lecture in Stockholm, 17 April 1912, GA 143.
21. Lecture in Berlin, 16 November 1908, GA 107.

22. Lecture in Dornach, 21 April 1924, GA 316.
23. Ibid.
24. Lecture in Dornach, 22 April 1924, GA 314.
25. Ibid.
26. Lecture in Dornach, 22 March 1920, GA 312.
27. Lecture in Dornach, 24 March 1920, GA 312.
28. Lecture in Dornach, 30 March 1920, GA 312.

2. Karma and Epidemics

29. Lecture in Stuttgart, 14 March 1906, GA 97.
30. Ibid.
31. Lecture in Berlin, 15 October 1906, GA 96.
32. Lecture in Hamburg, 18 May 1910, GA 120.
33. Ibid.
34. Lecture in Hamburg, 19 May 1910, GA 120.
35. Ibid.
36. Lecture in Hamburg, 22 May 1910, GA 120.
37. Lecture in Hamburg, 25 May 1910, GA 120.
38. Ibid.
39. 25 and 26 May 1910, GA 120.
40. Lecture in Hamburg, 26 May 1910, GA 120.

3. The Spiritual Background of Epidemics

41. Lecture in Dornach, 14 October 1917, GA 177.
42. Lecture in Dornach, 20 October 1918, GA 185.
43. Ibid.

4. Protection during Epidemics

44. Esoteric Lesson in Berlin, 1 November 1907, GA 266/1.
45. Lecture in Kassel, 9 May 1914, GA 261.
46. Ibid.
47. Ibid.
48. Ibid.
49. Ibid.

50. Ibid.
51. Lecture in Basel, 6 January 1920, GA 334.
52. Lecture in Dornach, 13 April 1921, GA 313.

5. Present Causes of Future Epidemics

53. Lecture in Paris, 2 June 1906, GA 94.
54. Lecture in Munich, 30 May 1907, GA 99.
55. Lecture in Kassel, 22 June 1907, GA 100.
56. Ibid.
57. Ibid.
58. Lecture in Munich, 14 June 1908, GA 98.
59. Ibid.
60. Ibid.
61. Ibid.
62. Ibid.
63. Ibid.

Items 11, 12, 14, 16, 26, 27 and 28 are taken direct from *Introducing Anthroposophical Medicine* (GA 312), translated by C. Creeger.

SOURCES

The following volumes are cited in this book. Where relevant, published editions of equivalent English translations are shown below the German titles.

The works of Rudolf Steiner are listed here (in brackets: date of the latest edition) with the volume numbers of the complete works in German, the *Gesamtausgabe* (GA), as published by Rudolf Steiner Verlag, Dornach, Switzerland.

RSP = Rudolf Steiner Press, UK
AP/SB = Anthroposophic Press / SteinerBooks, USA

57   *Wo und wie findet man den Geist?* (1984)
73a   *Fachwissenschaft und Anthroposophie* (2005)
94   *Kosmogonie* (2001)
      An Esoteric Cosmology (Garber Communications)
96   *Ursprungsimpulse der Geisteswissenschaft* (1989)
      Original Impulses for the Science of the Spirit (Completion Books, Australia)
97   *Das christliche Mysterium* (1998)
      The Christian Mystery (Completion Press)
98   *Natur- und Geistwesen—ihr Wirken in unserer sichtbaren Welt* (1996)
99   *Die Theosophie des Rosenkreuzers* (1985)
      Rosicrucian Wisdom (RSP)
100   *Menschheitsentwicklung und Christus-Erkenntnis* (2006)
107   *Geisteswissenschaftliche Menschenkunde* (1988)
120   *Die Offenbarungen des Karma* (1992)
      Manifestations of Karma (RSP)
127   *Die Mission der neuen Geistesoffenbarung* (1989)
143   *Erfahrung des Übersinnlichen. Die drei Wege der Seele zu Christus* (1994)

All English-language titles are available via Rudolf Steiner Press, UK (www.rudolfsteinerpress.com) or SteinerBooks, USA (www.steinerbooks.org)